Made in the USA
Middletown, DE
01 July 2021

43454722R00057